How to Heal Cavities and Reverse Gum Disease Naturally

Joey Lott

Copyright © 2017 Joey Lott

All rights reserved.

ISBN: **1542565685**
ISBN-13: **978-1542565684**

Contents

Preface 1

The Possibility of Healing Our Teeth 4

Dental Anatomy 7

Exploring Nutritional Building Blocks for Dental Health 10

Fat-Soluble Vitamins 12

Minerals 15

Demineralizing Substances 18

Protein 22

Metabolism 24

Diet 29

Circulatory Health 37

Supplements 40

Cleaning and Care 49

Toothpaste 50

Oil Pulling 53

What Now? 56

Get Another of My Books for Free 58

Please Write a Review of This Book 59

References 60

JOEY LOTT

Preface

Having strong, healthy teeth and gums is not merely a matter of chance. Neither is it merely a matter of brushing and flossing. And neither is it just a matter of lots of calcium, fluoride, vitamin D, or any of the other "magic bullet" solutions that we typically read about.

When you understand dental anatomy, metabolic factors, and basic nutritional information – none of which most of us ever learned – you too can improve the health of your teeth and gums.

Your gums and teeth are alive. They have the capacity to regenerate themselves (except, possibly, enamel).

Furthermore, as your oral health improves, you'll also likely discover that your overall health improves. Because your mouth is a part of your body, and its health reflects the overall health of your body.

Some of what you will learn in this book is congruent with the advice you're likely to hear elsewhere. For example, there are other, popular books on this subject that stress the importance of adequate fat-soluble vitamins for oral health. And in this book you'll learn again of this importance.

But much of what you will discover in this book may challenge what you think you know. For example, many of us have learned (incorrectly) that sugar (including fruit and fruit juice) causes cavities. This is not only not true, but this common advice to avoid sugar can actually be detrimental to your dental health. (No, I am not suggesting that you should start subsisting on candy and soda. Read on and you'll satisfy your curiosity on the subject.)

Please be prepared to read with an open mind. Unlike many other books on the subject, I provide references to scientific literature to back up my claims. And if you are willing to set aside what you think you know (that hasn't helped you), you'll find the information that I present to be logical, simple, and truthful.

This is a book about healing teeth naturally. That means that with the advice from this book, you may be able to regrow teeth (assuming the heart of the tooth is still intact), reduce or eliminate cavities, firm up loose teeth, and improve gum health.

None of this is science fiction.

As I've mentioned, there are other books on this subject, and there is also a good deal of information available for free on the internet on this subject. If you've read most of that other information, chances are, you've found it to be quite restrictive.

Typically, we are advised to adhere to rigid dietary protocols – typically low carbohydrate, high fat, "ancestral" diets. However, I am strongly of the (educated) opinion that such advice is unnecessarily restrictive and complicated. While it may work for some people some of the time, in the long run, it may do more harm than help if one can actually stick with the rigid protocols. More likely, most people simply will not or cannot manage such a restrictive approach to their lives and health. So in this book I offer a much more manageable approach to natural dental health that is free of much of the dogma found elsewhere.

In this book you'll learn how to use simple nutritional guidelines to provide a foundation for oral health. I'll first give you a primer on dental anatomy so that you can clearly see the logic and basis for the nutritional guidelines I offer.

Furthermore, I also suggest some additional lifestyle changes and practices that are proven to support good oral health.

If you're ready for a fresh, new perspective on natural dental healing that you can do yourself with an unrestrictive, enjoyable approach, then read on. You're in for a treat. I do not promise that you can get the same results as I did by applying the same principles, of course. However, I believe that the information in this book is some of the best on this subject.

The Possibility of Healing Our Teeth

We've all had the experience of looking at our teeth and thinking to ourselves, "Oh, it's really too bad that I've let my mouth go so far into disrepair since now I'll be stuck with these pitted, weakened, loose, and sensitive teeth and receding gums for the rest of my life."

And yet, what very few of us know is that our teeth and gums can heal. Although we receive a popular message quite to the contrary, anecdotal evidence from thousands of people around the world suggests that under the right conditions it often is possible to restore health to our teeth and gums.

That has been my own experience, and I have heard others report similar results. Many people seem to feel that they must follow a strict dietary protocol to achieve these results, yet I do not believe that this is necessary. I do believe that it is important to eat lots of nutrient-dense foods to support dental health. However, I do not believe that it is necessary to restrict one's diet to extremes as many others suggest.

Here is my experience: I followed many strict and pure dietary regimens over the years, many of which involved greatly restricting or eliminating sugars and starches as many experts suggest one should do. Yet in reality. my dental health declined slowly over the years. Due to extreme anxiety and other emotional problems that I experienced (and have written about elsewhere), I ended up neglecting my teeth for years. Because of this, I formed many cavities. In fact, one cavity on one of my wisdom teeth was so big that I could stick the tip of my tongue into it.

My teeth became very sensitive to just about everything. They hurt, and they became loose in the sockets as well. Like many people, I believed that what was done was done and there was nothing I could do about it.

However, when I put into practice the simple things that I outline in this book, I discovered that my teeth (and gums) began to heal. My teeth became less sensitive and firmed up in the sockets. My gums became healthier. They stopped bleeding and grew back up around the roots of the teeth from where they had receded. The cavities even began to fill back in. I didn't notice this until one day I tried to stick the tip of my tongue into that enormous cavity only to find that it had completely filled in with dentin!

In this book, I intend to share with you what I believe to be the easiest-to-follow guide on the subject of restoring health to teeth and gums through natural means. The information in this book is relatively inexpensive, easy to do, and sustainable. Furthermore, this is a simple guide, presented in a direct fashion. There's not a lot of fluff or confusing and unnecessary scientific-sounding filler. The science contained within this book is straightforward, relevant, and easy-to-understand.

Unlike other books, I see no need to make inflammatory claims against the dental industry or common dental practices. You are welcome to follow your dentist's suggestions if you wish. Nothing that I suggest in this book should be in conflict with your dentist's recommendations on a practical level, though your dentist may, of course, disagree with some of the claims that teeth can regrow. That is fine, though. Your dentist can disagree. You can follow the easy-to-do recommendations throughout the book, and you both can see what happens.

In other words, nothing in this book should be misconstrued as medical or dental advice, even though the subject of this book does deal with your health, including dental health. You are free to put into practice the ideas put forth in this book either independent of the advice of a dental professional or in conjunction with the advice of a dental professional. I have no desire to try and represent myself as a dental health expert. I'm just a normal person who happens to have researched these matters, tried a variety of extreme dietary protocols, and found some simple answers that have worked for me and for others. I hope that you find some benefit from what you read in this book as well.

Dental Anatomy

Our bodies are living. Just as your heart is alive, so too are your teeth alive. This may come as a surprise to you since we are often taught to think of our teeth as non-living structures, but when you look at the structure of teeth, you can see rather easily that they are, in fact, very much alive.

Now, to build a solid foundation of understanding, we're going to start by looking at the structure of teeth. This will be a little sciencey, but I'll keep it as simple as possible. So don't worry!

There are four major classifications of tissue that make up a tooth. Those are dental pulp, cementum, dentin, and enamel.

The dental pulp is a flesh-like tissue that connects the nerves and blood vessels from the rest of the body to the tooth. The pulp is at the core of the tooth, and the nerves and blood vessels pass through the roots of the teeth through the facial bones, and connect with the rest of the nervous and circulatory systems of the body. As long as the pulp is healthy, the rest of the tooth tissue can theoretically receive nutrition and other health-giving support from the rest of the body. Without the pulp, however, a tooth stands no chance of repairing itself.

The dentin tissue forms from the pulp, and it grows around the pulp. Dentin is composed primarily of mineral matter with a substantial amount of protein. Dentin is known to grow throughout the life of a tooth in response to various needs and stimuli. Dentin is thought to be necessary to support enamel.

Cementum is a mineralized tissue layer that forms around the dentin of the roots of a tooth. This tissue helps to connect a tooth to the socket. Specialized connective tissue called ligaments join the socket and the tooth by anchoring to the cementum.

Enamel is the hardest and most mineralized dental tissue. Enamel forms on the outer surface of the tooth above the gum line. Enamel is what allows us to chew relatively hard foods. Of course, due to the mineralized nature of enamel, it is also the most brittle type of dental tissue, as those of us who have chipped teeth can attest to. However, it is important to point out that while enamel has a high concentration of mineral content, it also contains some protein, which plays an important role in the living structure of enamel. So it is a mistake to think of enamel as a dead substance, because despite its hard structure, it is very much a living tissue.

The prevailing wisdom on the subject today seems to be that enamel does not regrow once it has been eroded. There have been some interesting studies in recent years that demonstrate the potential for stimulating enamel restoration, both through synthetic and natural means.

However, as of now, I don't know of any evidence that lead me to believe it is likely that most of us can regrow enamel that has gone missing. Good nutrition can strengthen existing enamel. But once enamel is gone from the surface of the tooth, don't expect it to regrow.

Still, restoring the health of your gums and teeth can do a great deal of repair, reduce symptoms, and improve the condition of your mouth – even if it doesn't result in regrowth of enamel.

In a nutshell, as long as the dental pulp remains, it is theoretically possible to restore health to a tooth. Most seem to agree that healthy dental pulp combined with good nutrition and oral health care can regrow dentin and strengthen existing enamel. In many cases, this may be enough to vastly improve dental health. Though dentists have various opinions on the matter, many find that it is possible to improve dental health through natural means to the extent that it is possible to avoid fillings and even root canals in some cases. I am not suggesting that this will be your experience. It may or it may not. However, anecdotally, many find this to be the case. Undoubtedly, at some point a dentist or two will write a scathing review of this book on the grounds that, in their opinion, it is reckless to suggest one might avoid a root canal. Yet again, anecdotally, many have reported good results with this approach for long periods of time. Ultimately, of course, the decision is yours - not mine, your dentist's, nor anyone else's.

Exploring Nutritional Building Blocks for Dental Health

Many times, experts from both mainstream and alternative perspectives tend to focus on minerals for dental health. For example, we've all heard the claims that topical fluoride can strengthen teeth, and we've surely all heard the marketing hype about the importance of calcium for strong teeth.

While minerals certainly do seem to play a very important role in dental health, it is a huge mistake to think that minerals alone are the sole key to healthy teeth.

Hopefully, you can already see why this would be. In the preceding section we saw how dental pulp is essential for tooth health, and this type of tissue has a very low mineral content. Unlike dentin, cementum, or enamel, pulp is fleshy and contains large amounts of nerve and capillary networks. Because the pulp is essential for tooth health, simply adding more minerals overlooks the importance of this central tooth tissue. Pulp requires metabolic health, nerve health, and circulatory health and depends on overall health.

Furthermore, while 70% of dentin is mineral content, the remaining 30% is organic tissue and water, which includes proteins. So while minerals are undoubtedly important for the health of dentin, that is only part of the picture. Adequate nutrition and overall health is essential for dentin health.

Even the highly-mineralized cementum and enamel contain some proteins and other organic materials. The cementum connects to the socket by way of ligaments, which are composed of proteins, so proper nutrition and health are necessary to support these tissues.

Hopefully, you can begin to see that good dental health isn't as overly simplistic as popping a calcium supplement and applying topical fluoride.

In the following sections, we'll explore some of the specific ways in which various aspects of nutrition can play an important role in dental health.

Fat-Soluble Vitamins

We've all heard of vitamins such as vitamin C or the B vitamin complex. Some of these vitamins are classified a water-soluble while others are classified as fat-soluble. While all vitamins may play an important role in dental health, the fat-soluble vitamins seem to play a particularly important role.

The fat-soluble vitamins include vitamins A, D, E, and K, and each of these vitamins is essential to overall health. Of these, A, D, and K seem to be the most important specifically for dental health.

Vitamin A is thought to be important for bone and tooth formation since it is involved in mineralization of some of the substances that make up bones and teeth. (Iwamoto, et al., 1994) Enamel contains some essential protein called keratin, which requires vitamin A for formation.

Typically, we are told that there are two types of vitamin A - carotenes (the orange and red pigments in vegetables such as carrots) and retinols (which are found only in animal foods). In reality, however, only retinols are true vitamin A. Theoretically, the human liver may be capable of converting carotenes into retinols, which is why carotenes are classified as vitamin A. However, not everyone converts carotenes well, so the only reliable sources of vitamin A are animal foods, of which liver seems to be the most potent source.

Vitamin D, which is more correctly classified as a hormone, is considered to be very important for bone and tooth health because it helps the body to absorb minerals. And at least one study found a remarkable reversal of tooth decay simply by adding supplemental vitamin D to the diets of the participants. (Mellanby & Pattison, 1932)

Many experts now claim that the majority of modern humans are deficient in vitamin D. Whether or not this is true, I cannot say. However, it is reasonable to understand how this might be so. Vitamin D is typically found in very small amounts in any food sources - animal and plant foods alike. Rather, the traditional source of vitamin D for humans is what the skin produces when exposed to sunlight. If naked humans living in tropical regions might be expected to form adequate vitamin D in this fashion, then it isn't hard to see how the average North American might be challenged in this regard.

Of course, humans have been clothed and living far away from the equator for a long time, so there must be traditional ways to increase vitamin D levels. It seems that sun exposure remains the tried and true means for increasing vitamin D levels, since adequate exposure during the warm months can theoretically raise levels sufficiently to carry one through the winter months. However, since most foods contain very small amounts of vitamin D, humans have also traditionally supplemented with high-vitamin specialty foods, such as cod liver oil, in regions where sunlight was a premium. (Don't worry, I'm not suggesting that you need to supplement with cod liver oil! We'll talk more about specific dietary and supplemental recommendations shortly.)

Finally, vitamin K is also thought to play an important role in tooth health. (Flore, et al., 2013) Vitamin K is really a group of similar compounds, and within the category there are two distinct types, which are called K1 and K2. K2 is the form that is thought to be used within the human body.

Vitamin K2 is thought to move minerals into the right places in the body – out of soft tissues and into bones and teeth. That makes K2 doubly important for tooth health, because for a tooth to be healthy, both the non-mineralized parts (the pulp) and the mineralized parts need to be working well. If the pulp is mineralized, then it will not function properly. Vitamin K2 helps keep the pulp free of excess minerals while keeping the dentin, cementum, and enamel mineralized.

K1 is found in plant sources, including many leafy greens. However, K1 from plant foods generally has poor bioavailability, though the bioavailability can be more than doubled with the addition of dietary fat to the same meal. Still, I wouldn't recommend depending on leafy greens as your primary source of vitamin K2 since the conversion rate from K1 to K2 is thought to be low.

K2 exists in animal foods as well as some specially-fermented foods in which bacteria produce K2. In fact, the food with the highest levels of K2 is natto, which is produced by bacterial fermentation of soy.

One last note regarding fat-soluble vitamins: since they are only soluble in fat, it is advisable to include adequate fat in one's diet. Without adequate dietary fat, it can be difficult for the body to properly metabolize the nutrients. What this means is that very low fat diets tend to lead to deficiencies in fat-soluble vitamins, which can adversely affect dental health.

Minerals

Although minerals are not the whole picture when it comes to dental health, they play an undeniably important role. Without adequate dietary minerals, it is all but impossible to enjoy good dental health.

When most people think of dental health, there are just two minerals that come to mind: fluoride and calcium. This oversimplification ends up being a detriment to many people's dental health, because dental health requires a lot more than just these two minerals.

To begin with, let me address fluoride. This is a very contentious issue, perhaps mostly due to the debate over water fluoridation. My personal preference is to avoid all supplemental fluoride. I live in a rural area with well water, and neither do I choose to use topical fluoride in toothpaste or otherwise. I personally do not feel that it makes sense for my own body. And, there is some good evidence that suggests that excessive fluoride exposure may have detrimental effects on the endocrine system, primarily impacting thyroid health, so I am glad to have no unnecessary fluoride exposure. (Navneet Singh, Verma, Verma, Sidhu, & Sachdeva, 2014) My dental health has increased significantly in the years since I have moved from cities in which I had fluoridated water, so in my view, supplemental fluoride doesn't seem to be helpful.

However, frankly, it is such a contentious political issue that I don't see the merit in taking a strong stance for the purposes of this book as I suspect that would distract from its value. Rather, I believe that the issue of fluoride is one that each individual must make. If you feel that supplemental fluoride is important for your dental health, then continue what you are doing. If you feel that supplemental fluoride is harmful to your health, and you prefer to avoid it, then do so. Either way, I believe that the information in this book can be helpful to you, and I don't see that supplemental fluoride will greatly help or hinder.

Though I will add this: the naturally-occurring form of fluoride that was originally shown to correlate to reduced cavity formation is calcium fluoride. Calcium reduces the toxicity of fluoride by as much as 43 times fluoride without calcium. The forms of fluoride added to water and otherwise used as supplements are not calcium fluoride. For what it's worth, I believe (but cannot prove) that adequate dietary calcium is *especially* important when ingesting fluoride from non-naturally-occurring sources.

With that out of the way, let's continue to look at the importance of minerals in terms of dental health.

Calcium certainly does seem to be an important mineral for tooth health. However, it is only one of the important minerals, and without the others in balance, calcium alone doesn't seem to be able to correct tooth problems. Furthermore, as indicated in the previous section, fat-soluble vitamins appear to be essential in terms of getting minerals, such as calcium, into teeth. So calcium without adequate fat-soluble vitamins doesn't seem to be very useful. In fact, without adequate fat-soluble vitamins, calcium and other minerals can end up in tissues, which can cause all sorts of health problems.

Weston A. Price was a dentist who is now famous (or infamous, depending on your view) for bringing to our attention the important role of nutrition in dental health. In his research there were significant differences in the diets of those who demonstrated good dental health versus those who demonstrate poor dental health. The two main differences that he found were between the levels of dietary fats and dietary minerals. In many cases, he found that those with good dental health ate approximately four times the minerals as those with poor dental health.

The minerals that are needed in the largest amounts are calcium, phosphorus, and magnesium. In addition, the body (and teeth) need all the trace minerals in smaller amounts. Of the trace minerals, those that are most significant for dental health include iron, copper, manganese, zinc, silica, and boron.

The good news is that as long as one eats enough quality, nutrient-dense food, then acquiring enough dietary minerals should not pose a problem. Neither does it need to require eating lots of "health" foods that no one enjoys eating. We'll take a look at this in more detail shortly.

Demineralizing Substances

Many drugs, both prescription and illicit, interfere with proper mineralization within the body. Drugs such as antibiotics, anticonvulsants, steroids, diuretics, and acid blockers are examples of types of drugs that can interfere with mineral absorption, so if you are using any of these drugs, then you may need to factor in the effect that these drugs may be having. (Cass, 2013)

Prescription drug use is at an all-time high. It is not likely to be a coincidence that many of the conditions and symptoms of those drugs are also at an all-time high. If you use prescription drugs and you are suffering from tooth decay or poor dental health, consider the impact that the drugs may be having. Obviously you should not discontinue any drugs without proper knowledge about the right way to do so – or if it is even safe or advisable to do so. But you may want to consider whether the drugs you take are actually necessary and whether you wish to continue taking them.

In addition, many foods include substances that interfere with mineral absorption. Some of the worst offenders are found in whole grains, legumes, nuts, seeds, and leafy green vegetables. A study that I referenced earlier found that regular consumption of oatmeal (a whole grain, rich in a substance that interferes with mineral absorption) in a vitamin D deficient diet was strongly correlated with tooth decay.

(Mellanby & Pattison, 1932) So the potential negative impacts of over-doing such foods shouldn't be overlooked.

Whole grains, legumes, nuts, and seeds contain substances known as anti-nutrients such as phytic acid that can bind to minerals and prevent their absorption. Phytic acid is a bound form of phosphorus, which is an important mineral for health. However, because the phosphorus is bound, it is not available for your body to use. Moreover, phytic acid can further bind to other minerals from other foods eaten at the same time, including phosphorus, calcium, magnesium, and so on.

In the previous edition of this book I suggested an overly-simplistic view of phytic acid. Basically, I implied that it is all bad – or at least undesirable. But I don't actually think that's true. I just think that it's perhaps a factor worth considering. If your diet is extremely high in phytic acid, you may need to increase your mineral intake or take other steps to compensate. Also keep in mind that in the study I referenced a few paragraphs ago, the researchers found that simply adding supplemental vitamin D to the diet reversed the tooth decay in the high-oatmeal diet participants.

Phytic acid may also have health benefits. It appears to have anti-cancer benefits and generally act as an antioxidant. (Fox & Eberl, 2002) So don't become paranoid about phytic acid. I'm sorry that I perpetuated the phytic acid fear to some extent in the original edition of the book. It's okay to relax about your food.

However, diets that are extremely high in phytic acid can have undeniably negative impacts on dental health *if you aren't taking some reasonable precautionary steps*. Namely, it is even more important that you eat plenty of minerals and fat-soluble vitamins.

In terms of where you'll find phytic acid, the primary sources are whole grains, nuts, seeds, and legumes. Phytic acid is the storage form of phosphorus, so it's no surprise that it's found in these foods – all of which are fundamentally seeds.

Traditionally many cultures that have relied heavily on these types of foods may have had processes for removing or reducing the phytic acid content. Those processes involve soaking, sprouting, leaching, peeling, and so forth.

A lot of contemporary "ancestral diet" proponents (at least those that even allow for the inclusion of such foods) recommend soaking and sprouting. I think it may be prudent to do so if you rely heavily on these foods and you are not also including other high mineral foods such as dairy. But to be honest, I think a lot of that stuff is excessive and unnecessary. I've had no problem eating plenty of foods high in phytic acid so long as I am also eating dairy and other sources of minerals.

Oxalic acid is another common anti-nutrient found in a variety of foods. The fact is that many foods contain oxalic acid, and so it is impossible to avoid. However, many of the foods that people commonly eat large quantities of in an attempt to be healthy actually contain huge amounts of oxalic acid. Some examples of foods with extremely high levels of oxalic acid include kale, spinach, and chard. There's nothing wrong with eating these foods in moderation, of course, and if you genuinely enjoy eating large amounts of raw kale and spinach every day, then take that as a sign that they are good for you. However, the practice of eating massive servings of these foods every day strictly out of ideological reasons may be misguided as the oxalic acid may bind to minerals, depleting stores in the body. Taste and cravings are probably the best indicators. If you crave raw spinach, then eat it. If not, then cramming it down anyway may not be a great idea.

With that said, the same points I made about phytic acid apply to oxalic acid. I haven't had problems with eating lots of oxalic acid so long as I am not relying on those foods for minerals. Also, there are gut bacteria that can degrade oxalic acid and liberate minerals. So at least in theory, if you are supporting healthy gut bacteria, you may actually be able to extract minerals from foods high in oxalic acid. So don't stress about eating oxalic acid either. Just be cognizant that spinach and so forth may not necessarily be the ideal source for minerals. And replacing entire meals with green smoothies may be misguided.

Protein

As we saw earlier, all of the tissues of the teeth require some essential protein in order to remain healthy. Strangely, protein is often overlooked as an important part of dental health, and yet without adequate quality protein, it is unreasonable to expect your teeth to be healthy.

In fact, some websites even suggest that one should cut down on protein as a strategy to keep teeth healthy. This is a misguided recommendation, however. While excessive dietary protein to the extreme is sure to have negative health consequences, it seems very unlikely that anyone other than bodybuilders and others who force themselves to eat extreme amounts of protein is likely to have a problem of too much protein.

More likely, however, is that most people are not eating protein with a good balance of amino acids. Many people are probably eating inflammatory proteins without a good balance of amino acids to nurture most of the body.

Think about this for a moment. Collagen is the most abundant protein in the human body. (Lodish, Berk, & Zipursky, 2000) As much as 57 percent of collagen is composed of the (anti-inflammatory) amino acid glycine, and human bones are made up of 25 percent glycine. (Eastoe, 1955) And yet modern humans eat almost no glycine.

Collagen isn't just important for bones. It's also important for joins, eyes, and organs such as the brain. Not surprisingly, it is also important for teeth. In fact, about 90% of the protein in dentin is composed of collagen. (Goldberg, Kulkarni, Young, & Boskey, 2011)

However, because most foods in the modern food system are deficient in collagen and/or some of the key amino acids that are found in collagen (such as glycine), you may not be getting enough of this important nutrient to support good health, including dental health. (We'll look at specific recommendations for how to remedy this in the Diet section.)

Also, although theoretically plant foods can supply a full array of amino acids, in practice this is very challenging for most people to achieve. Therefore, vegans may need to be especially careful in this regard. I was an ideological vegan for the better part of twenty years, and so I understand the ethical concerns of veganism, which are beyond the scope of this book to address (though I have covered the matter in my book, *Vegan Recovery*). However, if your teeth aren't doing so great on a vegan diet, then there may be dietary issues undermining your dental health. These issues can include anti-nutrients, lack of fat-soluble vitamins, too little energy (calories), insufficient minerals, or poor quality or inadequate protein.

Metabolism

Now that we've looked at the major building blocks for dental health, we're almost ready to take a look at some specific dietary recommendations. However, before we jump to that, there is one more very important factor that consider, and that is the role of metabolism in dental health.

I believe that metabolism is the big missing piece for many people's health. I am passionate about this subject because when I finally caught on to this (along with the incredibly important role that stress plays in health), I began to turn around major health problems that had been plaguing me for years, including chronic fatigue, chronic Lyme disease, major insomnia, and some other problems that were negatively impacting my quality of life.

I also personally found metabolism to be a key component of improving my dental health, which is a connection I believe few people understand.

Metabolism means the production of energy from nutrients such as sugar (glucose) or fat. Everything in the body is governed by how healthy the metabolism is. That's not surprising if you think about it; after all, every cell in your body needs energy!

While there are many possible factors that can determine metabolic health, one of the surest ways to harm metabolism is by chronically undereating.

Strange as it may seem, I find that many people nowadays are undernourished, even if they are eating a lot of volume. This is true both of people who are eating lots of fast food and industrial junk food *and* people who are trying to each "healthy".

That people overeating junk food would be undernourished shouldn't come as a big surprise. Although I staunchly defend the value of all natural foods, including refined sugar and flour in the context of a diet and lifestyle that is well-balanced, I certainly don't advocate for excessive consumption of Big Macs and Coca-Cola. Highly-processed industrial food stuffs often contain little in the way of minerals or essential vitamins and can contain artificial ingredients, preservatives, and other undesirables.

But it may come as a surprise to discover that people who are trying to eat healthfully could be undernourished. After all, shouldn't all the brown rice and salads or the low-carb variant of steamed kale and bone broth add up to super nutrition? Yet it seems that the healthier people try to eat, the greater the risk of under-nourishment. The reason is because a healthy metabolism requires a consistent input of food energy - also known as calories.

Not surprisingly, the extremes cause problems while the middle ground offers the most desirable results. We need plenty of vitamins and minerals *and* we need plenty of calories. The junk food diet offers calories in abundance with little in the way of other nutrients. On the other hand, the extremes of "health food" are typically short on calories and, depending on the principals one adheres to, may be short on some key nutrients as well (vegan diets are notorious for being deficient in bioavailable minerals and quality protein as well as some key B vitamins, for example, while low carb diets are too low in [surprise, surprise] carbohydrates).

The truth is that to do proper justice to the subject of metabolism and the role that under-eating can play in harming metabolism would require another book. Necessarily, in this book I am going to leave a lot out of the discussion of metabolism. However, much of the necessary discussion for explaining this subject is only required because many of us are convinced that the only "healthy" diets are those that (often indirectly) involve calorie restriction. As such, it often requires a great deal of convincing to explain to people that all the theories of healthy diets are meaningless unless a person is eating enough calories.

Truly, the facts are rather simple. While many of the diets that are promoted as ideal (such as whole foods, vegan, raw vegan, paleo, low carb, etc.) have convincing-sounding arguments, what most all of them leave out is that if one isn't getting enough energy from food (i.e. calories), then no amount of antioxidants or "life-force" or anything else will make up for that in terms of your basic needs. And in the face of a sustained calorie deficit, the body will slow metabolism.

Slowed metabolism has lots of symptoms associated with it, including:

- insomnia or disturbed sleep (often waking in the early morning with symptoms of high cortisol and/or adrenaline)
- depression
- anxiety
- food sensitivities or intolerances
- leaky gut
- irritable bowel
- edema or fluid retention
- intolerance to cold (and sometimes heat)
- cold hands and feet
- low or non-existent sex drive
- memory and/or cognitive problems
- dry skin, possibly rashes
- muscle and joint pain
- falling hair
- weight gain or weight loss (weight gain is more typical, but weight loss can result, particularly in chronic hypometabolic cases when a person has difficulty consuming enough food)
- frequent urination - particularly at night

- fatigue

If you experience any of those symptoms and/or your temperature is consistently less than 98.6 degrees Fahrenheit (37 degrees Celsius) or your resting pulse is under 65 beats per minute, then you likely have a slowed metabolic rate. Also, if your thyroid hormone levels are low (resulting in a slowed metabolism), you should consider the possibility that the actual cause is under-eating, since under-eating has consistently been shown to lower thyroid hormone levels. (Lott, Big Fat Lies, 2015)

A slowed metabolism means that your whole body's health will be compromised, including dental health. Remember that dental health isn't just about minerals. It also involves living tissue that is connected with the rest of the body. If your metabolism is slowed and therefore your body isn't functioning optimally, then that will make it very difficult for your teeth to be healthy.

If you are eating too little, then it will be all but impossible to improve your metabolism.

When I first learned of how much healthy weight-stable people eat, I was shocked. I had been accustomed to eating far less than that. And it also easily explained part of why I felt so terrible.

When healthy, weight-stable people are studied to find out how much they actually eat (versus how much they report), it turns out that pregnant and lactating women of all ages, as well as men under the age of 25, eat 3500 calories a day. Men aged 25 and over, as well as women under the age of 25, eat 3000 calories a day. And women who are neither pregnant nor lactating and who are aged 25 or over eat 2500 calories a day.

So, if you have a slowed metabolism and you are eating less than those figures and you aren't feeling so great, then you might want to consider eating more. There are no guarantees, of course. However, anecdotally, I'm far from the only one who has experienced health benefits from eating more, and those health benefits have included improvements in dental health.

I do understand that you may have reservations about eating more. Most people do, especially because most people seem to be convinced that they are too fat. Yet I encourage you to set aside what you think you know about these things, and instead ask your body what you need. If your body needs more energy, then you might consider that your ideological diets have not been helping you.

Diet

Almost all of the popular advice for how to improve dental health through nutrition ends up being unnecessarily restrictive, in my opinion. It seems that almost universally everyone who offers nutritional advice for dental health demonizes sugar, and then many of the advocates of traditional diets (such as the Weston A. Price Foundation) suggest that even many natural sugars are problematic. Many will even go so far as to recommend that one eliminates carbohydrates (except fiber, of course) entirely!

In my own experience this is not only unnecessary, but it can sometimes be harmful. This is why the diet that I recommend is much more lenient than most of what you'll find elsewhere.

I *do* believe that it is sensible and wise to stick to real foods that are as nutrient-dense as possible - within reason. And, there are some important caveats, as we'll explore together. So I'm not suggesting that it is necessarily advisable to eat a diet consisting of nothing more than Twinkies, Lifesavers, and chocolate chip cookies, but neither does it seem advisable to me to swing to the extreme of eliminating all sugar and all refined starches and only ever eating cod liver oil, high vitamin butter oil, and kale, as it would seem some suggest.

I believe there is a sensible, practical, and sustainable middle ground. This involves what I call "intuitive eating" coupled with an awareness of eating enough to support metabolic health and some suggestions for foods to try to include regularly. This doesn't have to be a rigid diet. In fact, it is best if it is not(!), because a rigid diet isn't usually sustainable.

Furthermore, my suggestions are actually in line with some of the findings that Dr. Price reported in his book, *Nutrition and Physical Degeneration*. In that book, he reported that he recorded improvements in dental health of children who received a single supplementary meal daily in which they ate cod liver oil and high-vitamin butter oil (the combination supplying vitamins A, D, and K2) along with a quality meat broth (supplying collagen). Even though these children were otherwise still eating the same diets that had led to tooth decay, this simple supplementation resulted in dental health improvements.

So it does not seem to me that it is necessary or even desirable to radically change one's diet in a restrictive fashion as many modern health proponents suggest we should. My observation is that many, if not most, people who do so end up with worse health problems than when they started the restrictive diet. The deterioration may take months or it may take years. However, I see it happen time and time again. I believe there is a better way.

The following are my recommendations for a better way.

There are two basic guidelines to the diet that I recommend:

1. One must eat enough (see guidelines for adequate daily calories from previous section) from a variety of foods, including all macronutrients (fat, protein, and carbohydrates).

2. One must eat enough nutrient-dense foods to supply adequate vitamins and minerals.

In practice, this is pretty easy to do. Or, I should say, it is theoretically easy to do, and once one gets the hang of it, it is very easy to do. However, the biggest challenge that most people have is that they refuse to comply with the first guideline because they are adhering to a restrictive diet because of ideology or out of fear. That is typically the biggest hurdle.

Here is where I tell you that my dental health improved dramatically when I started eating massive amounts of sugar and dramatically increasing my caloric intake from an average of around 1600 calories a day to an average of 3500 calories per day.

Why would eating so much sugar help my dental health? I don't know for certain, but I suspect it has a lot to do with metabolism. Eating a lot of sugar helped me to fuel a healthy metabolism because I was supplying adequate calories and carbohydrates. Until that happens, it is darn near impossible to sustain good health, including dental health. Does that mean that there aren't people who live off of a 1600 calorie a day diet with absolutely no sugar and have stellar dental health? Of course not. Never say never. There may be some people who manage that, but I wasn't one of them. And you probably aren't either. The vast majority of evidence suggests you need a lot of calories and a lot of nutrients.

My experience and the experiences of many others I have communicated with on this subject is that it is very difficult (as in, almost impossible) to eat enough to fuel a healthy metabolism *and* stick to a "perfect" and "healthy" diet, such as raw vegan or low carb paleo. That doesn't mean that it is strictly impossible, of course. Some people might be able to do it, but it is extremely difficult if not impossible. So my finding is that eating *enough* is more important than eating only the "right" foods.

Once you're eating enough, you can start to try to eat enough while only eating the "right" foods if that still feels important to you, but in my experience, getting the metabolism functioning is the most important first step.

I personally got my metabolism working more optimally by eating massive amounts of easy-to-digest energy sources, including lots of whole dairy, butter, sugar, white rice, potatoes, and fruit juice. Of course, apart from the milk and butter, these foods are usually what the "experts" tell us are the worst for dental health. Yet, I found exactly the opposite, and I'm not alone.

Really, I believe that a lot of well-intentioned people today are placing unnecessary restrictions on their diets and suggesting that others do the same simply because they are basing their advice on ideologies that they never actually tested themselves. Dr. Price found that adding in nutrient-dense "superfoods" was sufficient to improve dental health in children. He didn't report that the children had to eliminate all grain and all sugar. And this is consistent with my own experience. In fact, my dental health deteriorated during the times when I eliminated all grain and all sugar, and it improved when I added grain and sugar back into my diet. I believe this is largely because of metabolic health and not because of the particular foods.

Others may find that their dental health improves when they remove all sugar from their diet, but this may be coincidental. The elimination of sugar may not have caused the improvement in dental health. It may have been other factors, such as including more nutrient-dense foods or more fat-soluble vitamins.

In practice, I find that *enough* food is far more important than the ideologically correct food.

The second guideline is to eat enough nutrient-dense food to supply the necessary vitamins and minerals to improve dental health. This seems to be just as important as the first guideline.

In practice, it seems that the most important foods are quality fats and high-mineral foods as well as enough balanced proteins. Some of the real superstar foods here include the following:
- Butter
- Coconut oil
- Whole milk and other dairy foods
- Collagen-rich foods/gelatin
- Egg yolks
- Organ meats - particularly liver from grass-fed ruminants
- Mineral-rich salt

As I have stated repeatedly, I have eaten a lot of sugar (evaporated sugar cane juice – both with and without the molasses) as part of my dental recovery. But in addition to eating sugar, I also eat lots of nutrient-dense foods. I drink lots of whole milk (I have a preference for raw milk when possible, though I'm not convinced that it is necessary that milk be raw as many people claim – I just prefer the taste). I eat lots of butter. I eat lots of egg yolks. I eat a lot of gelatin. And I frequently eat liver and other organ meats.

I believe that these foods really do improve dental health.

Some people claim that they have intolerances to dairy. Anecdotally, however, dairy - especially whole milk - does tend to be very useful for improving dental health. It contains a lot of minerals that are hard to find from other common foods. It also contains valuable quality fats, so it's worth making a few notes on this subject.

As I detailed in my book, *Food Myths*, many people mistakenly believe they cannot tolerate dairy because of lactose. It is true that approximately 70 percent of the world's human population does not have the genetic variation that causes them to produce the enzyme that breaks down lactose into adulthood. *However*, in those cases lactose acts like fiber in the gut, and bacteria in the digestive system can digest the milk sugar.

Until one builds up the bacterial populations in the gut, it's not a great idea to eat a large amount of milk or lactose-containing dairy. The result will be digestive distress – much the same as suddenly doubling your dietary fiber intake could lead to digestive distress. However, slowing increasing dairy over many weeks or months can alleviate the problem. And as an added bonus, for those without the lactose-digesting enzyme, building up dairy tolerance will also build a healthier gut microbiome, improving immune health.

Many people promote bone broth as being a good sources of minerals. And I even reported the same in the first edition of this book. However, it turns out that is not true. Bone broth is not a great source of minerals. What it is a great source of is gelatin. So if you're inclined to make and consume bone broth, it has plenty of health benefits. But minerals don't appear to be one of them (except, perhaps, some toxic metals – more on that later).

So if you're not going to consume dairy, I think it's important to find other good sources of minerals. As I reported in my book *Food Myths*, leafy green vegetables are not a good enough source of calcium, despite being touted as such. Apart from dairy, the only other excellent source of calcium of which I am aware is small, whole fish with bones in (such as sardines). Supplemental minerals may be necessary for those who avoid dairy and aren't eating calcium-rich foods such as bone-in sardines regularly.

While many "experts" claim that one should eat *only* nutrient-dense whole foods, I don't believe this is necessary or even necessarily helpful. As I indicated earlier, Dr. Price reported that simply *adding* nutrient-dense foods to existing diets of some populations resulted in improvement in dental health. This is consistent with my own findings, so I caution against becoming fanatical about eating *only* nutrient-dense whole foods, because in practice it can backfire and work against you.

Or, another way to think of it is this: calories are an essential nutrient. And so when you are choosing "nutrient-dense" foods, be sure to also factor in the importance of calories. From that perspective, kale isn't sufficiently nutrient-dense to cover all your needs. Kale may be part of a nutrient-dense diet. But so might be sugar and white flour and fruit juice if you need the calories.

In the original edition of this book I had a third guideline. That guideline was to avoid toxins and anti-nutrients. In this revision of the book I decided to downplay the importance of this factor, and it is no longer one of the guidelines. But it is still a point worth discussing.

When possible, it is ideal to eat food grown or raised without chemical pesticides or fertilizers and without added drugs, as are often added to conventionally-raised animals. When buying packaged foods, look for those without any chemical additives.

Why? Because some of those pesticides, drugs, and chemical additives can bind to minerals and disrupt hormones.

I don't think it's something you need to become fanatical about. Don't become paranoid and afraid of eating food. But it will probably be beneficial to eat *primarily* fresh (not overly processed, packaged) foods that are produced without the use of lots of drugs or chemicals.

In some places like the United States some of the persistent pesticides like lindane and DDT are banned for agricultural use, and levels in food (and human bodies) have dropped significantly since then. But because they are still in use in other parts of the world and because they are persistent for many decades, they are still found in many foods in the food supplies, even in places where the chemicals are banned.

The highest levels are found in ocean fish and other seafood. Farmed fish is even worse – containing 10 times the levels of contaminants of wild fish. So I think it is wise to limit seafood and to completely avoid farmed fish. (Small fish such as sardines may be the exception because they generally won't have picked up as many contaminants as larger fish. And I do eat a lot of sardines and oysters, as a matter of fact.)

As for anti-nutrients, I think the concerns raised by many fad diet proponents are overstated – even though in the first edition of this book I recommended caution when it comes to high levels of phytates or oxalic acid.

Let me be clear: I do not believe there is convincing evidence that it makes sense to be paranoid about modest amounts of phytates or oxalic acid. Eating some whole grain bread, brown rice, spinach, kale, etc., isn't a problem....*so long as* you are eating sufficient amounts of mineral-rich foods. And despite what you may read in the internet or in vegan propaganda, whole grains, beans, and green vegetables are *not* good sources of minerals because the minerals are bound up and not bioavailable.

With that said, please also keep in mind that eating excessive amounts of those foods – whole grains, beans, green vegetables, etc. - will result in mineral deficiencies. So if you're eating green smoothies and oatmeal and brown rice for every meal, you're not setting yourself up for successful tooth mineralization.

Many people want to be purists and eat only sprouted whole grains (since sprouting reduces the anti-nutrient content of grains, beans, nuts, and seeds). This is fine, of course. However, many people end up with a calorie deficit when they do this, so if you have a slowed metabolism, then I encourage you to consider focusing on improving metabolic health *first* before trying to be a purist.

The other "anti-nutrient" worth considering is polyunsaturated oils such as canola, soy, corn, and safflower. While small amounts of polyunsaturated fat seem to be fine, large amounts work as a metabolism suppressant. Some types of saturated fat, on the other hand, appear to have a beneficial effect on metabolism. In particular, butyric acid and lauric acid, which are found in butter and coconut oil, respectively, are fatty acids that are shown to have pro-metabolic activity. So for what it's worth, you'll probably get the best results by ditching so-called "vegetable" oils (seed oils high in omega 6 polyunsaturated fatty acids) and replacing them with small amounts of butter and coconut oil as well. Olive oil is also modestly pro-metabolic.

Overall, hopefully you can begin to see how the guidelines work together to outline a diet that can be inclusive, enjoyable, sustainable, and healthy. Very little in this diet is excluded. In fact, nothing is strictly excluded (though I really would recommend you avoid farmed fish as much as possible). Rather, the first and most important guideline is that you must eat enough. Then, I suggest that you include some foods that most people find to be delicious and enjoyable. For example, butter and collagen-rich broth tend to improve the flavor of most foods. And then finally, there are just a few ideas for ways to minimize unnecessary toxins and anti-nutrients so as to maintain hormonal and mineral balance.

It is not advisable to be neurotic or fanatical about any of this. In fact, trying to be a purist just produces stress, which undermines health. I honestly believe it is best to enjoy a stress-free diet that includes lots of delicious and palatable foods. Let your appetite be your guide. Eat delicious food. Enjoy what you eat. Have no restrictions based on ideology, which means you shouldn't restrict foods based on anything in this book, either. Rather, just *don't force* yourself to eat or to restrict anything because you think it is healthy.

Circulatory Health

As I mentioned earlier, dental health depends in part on the health of the circulatory system. This is true not only of gums, but also of teeth. And it is worth keeping in mind that dental health is often viewed as an indicator of cardiovascular health, perhaps because dental health will suffer if the health of the cardiovascular system is suffering.

Cardiovascular health is, rightfully so, a hot topic these days. After all, 1 in 4 people will die of cardiovascular disease.

But most people have been taught that the main causes of cardiovascular disease are saturated fat and cholesterol. That turns out to be misleading and generally unhelpful. After all, in the time during which populations have been convinced to significantly reduce their saturated fat and cholesterol intake as well as take cholesterol-lowering drugs (statins are the most prescribed drugs in the world), cardiovascular disease has continued to increase.

Not only has the conventional advice failed to help most people reduce their real cardiovascular disease risk. It also steers people away from important dietary sources of nutrients for overall health and particularly for dental health — foods such as full-fat dairy and eggs.

Fortunately, new research indicates that inflammation and inadequate nutrition may underlie many cardiovascular problems. And certainly there is evidence that both of these causes are likely to be factors in dental health problems. So let's take a look at what factors can support cardiovascular/circulatory health in terms of inflammation and nutrition.

Nutritional factors that are shown to improve endothelial health (meaning the lining of the circulatory system) include vitamin C, (Ashor, Lara, Mathers, & Siervo, 2014) bioflavonoids, and polyphenols. (Grassi, et al., 2013)

In practical terms, these things are found primarily in fruits, vegetables, and herbs.

These same nutrients also reduce inflammation.

Some of the most potent common food/herb sources of these nutrients include: coffee, green tea, turmeric, blueberries, raspberries, blackberries, and strawberries.

But don't stop there. Plenty of other fruits and vegetables and herbs are great sources of these nutrients. Include citrus, citrus peels, oregano, ginger, potatoes, carrots, and so forth in your diet.

In addition to diet, lifestyle factors also play an important role in circulatory health.

Exercise has gotten a lot of attention in the popular press. And it's true that moderate exercise has many proven benefits for cardiovascular health.

Over-exercise has *negative* impacts, however. It increases stress and inflammation, and produces cardiovascular damage.

So moderation is key. If you're running for an hour or more a couple times a week, you're probably overdoing it. But if you're sitting around all the time, you're underdoing it.

One of the best and safest forms of exercise, not surprisingly, is walking. And unless you walk vigorously for many hours every day, you'd have a hard time overdoing it.

To get the best benefits from walking, do it outside. Because another lifestyle factor involved in cardiovascular health is sunlight. Getting regular sunlight exposure – unfiltered through windows – is also proven to have cardiovascular benefits. (Holick, 2002)

And finally, another important lifestyle factor for cardiovascular health (which will support dental health) is adequate sleep. Studies show that inadequate sleep is strongly associated with cardiovascular disease. (Lott, 2014) Most people need around 8 hour of sleep, give or take an hour. How much you need is entirely individual. So sleep as much as you need every night. It's good for your heart and it's good for your teeth and gums. Don't underestimate the importance of sleep. Really. It's a big deal.

Supplements

The idealists among us may want to achieve perfect health without any supplements whatsoever. This is fine except that it usually doesn't work. I find that some good quality supplements are really helpful in this regard.

However, unlike many of the self-proclaimed experts who write on this subject of natural dental health, I do not personally believe that it is necessary or even helpful to rely on super expensive and "pure" supplements.

Dr. Price studied the effects of supplementing diets with cod liver oil as well as high-vitamin butter oil, which is made by centrifuging the spring butter from grass-fed cows. He found very favorable results with these two supplements. As a result, most "experts" now recommend that people supplement with cod liver oil and high-vitamin butter oil.

There are a few problems with this, however. For one thing, these two supplements are very expensive. And for another thing, they don't always work for people. In fact, some people react badly to cod liver oil.

Dr. Price himself warned of the negative health effects of poor quality cod liver oil, and there is good reason to believe that most, if not all, cod liver oil on the market would fit the definition of poor quality cod liver oil given by Dr. Price.

What most people do not realize is that almost *all* cod liver oil on the market has been molecularly distilled to remove contaminants *and that process also removes the natural vitamins*. So with only a few exceptions, cod liver oil you can buy has synthetic vitamins added to it rather than the natural vitamins from the cod liver oil, meaning you're better off just taking the (synthetic) vitamins directly rather than the (more expensive and possibly rancid) cod liver oil with the vitamins added.

As of this writing there are only three cod liver oil products available to a broad market that are *not* molecularly distilled. One is fermented. Two are not.

Recently there was a big drama within the Weston A. Price Foundation "community" in which people became divided on the issue of fermented versus non-fermented cod liver oil. There was money at stake and the major players in the drama all stood to profit.

But what was not brought to light during that drama was this: none of the three cod liver oil products that are being promoted as containing naturally-occurring vitamins are proven to be safe.

The companies selling those products claim that they do routine testing for their products to ensure there are no contaminants. But when I contacted the companies, requesting the test results for specific batches/lots of their products, not one provided adequate documentation.

Foods from the ocean stand a very high likelihood of being contaminated with dangerous chemicals and toxic metals, including DDT, mercury, lead, arsenic, PCBs, and so forth. These are not things you want to be eating much of. And foods from the ocean routinely test dangerously high in these chemicals and metals.

Fish oil that has been properly molecularly distilled will not have dangerous levels of these contaminants. But fish out that has *not* been molecularly distilled almost certainly will. And I do not think it is unreasonable as a consumer to demand from sellers that they supply third party test results on their products. In fact, in many food and supplement niches it is standard practice that any customer who makes a request will receive a certificate of analysis with third party test results matching the specific lot or batch the customer has purchased or is considering purchasing.

But as I said, none of the three companies selling natural cod liver oil supply adequate documentation on request.

I would not personally eat any of their cod liver oil products for that reason.

While it is usually a mistake to try and reduce a food to vitamin or mineral components, nonetheless, I suspect that much of the benefit of these supplemental foods is due to the fat-soluble vitamin content. As such, I believe that it is possible to obtain the same benefits (if not greater benefit) at less cost and with greater ease with a few simple and inexpensive supplements combined with real, nutrient-dense food.

I believe that cod liver oil is traditionally valued primarily because it is a rich source of both vitamin A and vitamin D in an ideal ratio (approximately 5:1). And I believe that high-vitamin butter oil is traditionally valued because it is a rich source of vitamin K2.

Personally, I have benefited from local, grass-fed lamb liver for vitamin A and supplemental vitamins D and K. I have also taken supplemental vitamin A in the retinyl palmitate form.

Chris Masterjohn wrote an excellent article that is published on the Weston A. Price Foundation's website that describes why synthetic vitamin A is likely okay and why the ratio between vitamins A and D is so important. (Masterjohn, 2006) He provides a lot of references showing that high levels of vitamin A – even from natural sources – without adequate vitamin D result in bone (and tooth) mineral loss. But in a ratio of approximately 5:1 to 8:1, vitamins A and D from food or supplements provide support for health, including bone and tooth health, even in very large amounts.

Vitamin D has gotten a lot of hype in recent years. And so, not surprisingly, there's also been a lot of backlash. So you can easily find groups claiming that vitamin D is the greatest thing for health under the sun. But you can also easily find plenty of people claiming that supplemental vitamin D is dangerous and will cause heart attacks and kidney stones.

Who to believe?

I don't know. But what I can tell you is that I personally don't worry about it. I take the approach of keeping fat soluble vitamins – particularly A, D, and K – in balance.

Vitamin D is said to increase calcium (and magnesium) absorption. So in theory, if a person gets a lot of vitamin D from any source (including from sun exposure) and eats a lot of calcium *and* has a vitamin K2 deficiency, a lot of calcium could possibly get deposited into soft tissues, resulting in a heart attack or kidney stones. And, in fact, I read a report that lifeguards statistically have higher rates of kidney stones than the rest of the population – possibly because of higher levels of vitamin D.

But in theory, vitamin K2 moves calcium out of soft tissues and into bones and teeth. And in theory, that will eliminate the danger.

I have personally gotten positive results from a daily vitamin D/K combination liquid supplement. I have found that the Thorne liquid D/K combination works really well for me. (I have no affiliation with Thorne.) There are likely other good quality liquid D and K products. I can only recommend Thorne because that is the one that I have personally found to be useful.

When you are looking for D and K, I recommend a liquid in oil that is not soy oil. Good oil bases are usually olive oil or medium chain triglycerides, which is derived from coconut or palm oil. Also, look for products that have limited or no additional ingredients. The Thorne product I use has added tocopherols, which are vitamin E added presumably as an antioxidant. Some products contain weird chemical additives, and I would steer clear of them since I don't know what those additives do.

Most literature that I have read on vitamin D suggests that D3 is the preferable form (though many say it makes no difference whether it is D2 or D3), and it is safe to take at least 4000 IU daily. There is a lot of scary advice to avoid taking "too much" vitamin D because of the potential for overdose. However, upon actually examining this, it turns out that overdose seems to be difficult to achieve. I have read of some accidental overdoses in which people were unknowingly taking over 200,000 IU a day for months (because of a manufacturer error) before noticing symptoms. Discontinuing supplementation resolved those problems from what I have read. Standard recommendations range from 2000 IU to 4000 IU a day, and these seem to be safe. I'm no expert on the matter. However, I've read quite a lot on the subject, and if you want to be conservative, then 2000 IU to 4000 IU seems to be the right range for daily supplementation. And since vitamin D is fat-soluble, you can also take larger amounts less frequently, if you prefer. For example, you could take 14,000 IU once a week, which would be the equivalent of 2000 IU daily.

But based on Chris Masterjohn's research, I now make sure that my vitamin A and vitamin D intake is in the 5:1 to 8:1 range. So if I eat or supplement with 25,000 IU of vitamin A, I will supplement with 3,000-5,000 IU vitamin D (assuming I'm not out in the sun with few clothes on for a few hours, that is).

Vitamins A and D have some antagonistic properties, and taking an excess of one can effectively deplete the other. Vitamin D is the darling of so many health "experts" these days, and so I believe many people are supplementing far in excess of vitamin D without the balance of vitamin A. As a result, many people are likely vitamin A deficient, and their health suffers as a consequence.

From what I have read about vitamin K, the recommendations are all over the place. However, it does seem reasonable to supplement with K2 (versus K1) since it would seem to be the form that the body prefers. The reports that I have read so far suggest that there is no actual upper limit with vitamin K2. It doesn't seem to be toxic, even in very large doses assuming you use the MK-4 (menatretenone) form. I don't see the sense in being extreme, though. I have actually taken large doses (45 mg daily) without noticing any particular benefit. And so for the money, I prefer to just take the Thorne D/K liquid, which supplies 200 mcg per 1000 IU of D. Therefore, if I take 2000 IU of D, then I get 400 mcg of K2 or if I take 5000 IU of D, then I get 1000 mcg (1 mg) of K2. This works just as well for me as taking the large amounts of K. (Actually, it's more economical to use the Thorne K2 supplement and D3 supplement separately. But it's easier to take the D/K combination supplement.)

For vitamin A, I eat a fair amount of liver plus a lot of eggs (yolks) and some butter. (I used to eat a lot more butter (averaging 1 stick of butter per day), but have less desire for it in recent years, and I haven't noticed any health problems reducing the amount of butter I eat [to probably half what I used to eat].) I also eat foods with pro-vitamin carotenes and lycopenes and so forth (chard, carrots, sweet potatoes, tomatoes, watermelon, etc.), which may get converted to vitamin A as needed – though also may not, since some people are not good converters. Also, in recent times, I've added a vitamin A supplement in the form of retinyl palmitate since reading the Chris Masterjohn article I mentioned earlier. I am inconsistent about it, but make take anywhere from 25,000 to 100,000 IU in a day when I think to do so and am not eating liver that day.

Keep in mind that preformed vitamin A (retinol from liver, egg yolks, butter, etc. or retinyl from retinyl palmitate) is kind of controversial. There is a popular belief that consistently eating more than maybe 5,000 IU per day will lead to vitamin A toxicity. So don't follow my lead regarding vitamin A if you aren't educated on the matter and willing to buck the conventional wisdom.

However, personally, at present I am not concerned about eating what probably amounts to something in the range of 25,000 IU of preformed vitamin A per day *so long as* I get about 1/8th or so (by IU) as much vitamin D. And I'm not concerned about the amount of vitamin D I consume or produce so long as I get enough vitamins A and K2.

Another supplemental food that I really like, and one that I believe has helped me tremendously, is gelatin. Gelatin is a protein produced from collagen, and so gelatin is a really convenient way to eat more of this really important and nourishing protein. And as I have stated previously, collagen is the most abundant protein in the human body, including in the teeth, so eating gelatin is a really simple and easy way to provide this important nutrient.

Since collagen is the most abundant protein in most animals, then the traditional practice of eating the entire animal ensured adequate dietary collagen. However, in the modern food system, most of us have little access to the collagen-rich parts of the animal. While we usually can find bones to make into collagen-rich bone broth, this takes a lot of time that many of us simply don't have, so gelatin is a convenient alternative.

I purchase beef gelatin from a company called Great Lakes. A natural food store in my area carries it, but if you cannot find it locally in your area, you can find it on the internet. In fact, there is currently a vendor selling it on Amazon.com for less than the local natural foods store's price, so you can find it at very reasonable prices online if you look. Other companies also sell gelatin (NOW Foods, for example), which may be of excellent quality as well. I simply cannot personally attest to it.

A popular fad these days is bone broth. I do believe that bone broth is a nutritious traditional food with many possible health benefits. But surely one of those benefits – if not the primary benefit – is gelatin. I find that cooking bone broth is more than I am realistically going to manage on a regular basis. So for me, Great Lakes gelatin is a good alternative. Also, keep in mind that animals store lead in the bones. That makes bone broth a pretty good source of lead – not something you want to eat a lot of. I don't know the exact levels of lead in bone broth, but I have read some studies that show that lead levels in bones today are about 8 times higher than they were a few hundred years ago. So it *may* be that gelatin from hides (like Great Lakes) is a safer source of gelatin than bone broth for daily use.

In the previous edition of this book I recommended calcium bentonite clay as a good source of dietary minerals. I even said that I believed that it was one of the best things I had done for my teeth.

Now I am not so sure. It's hard to get good information on the subject as to whether bentonite clay is actually a good source of minerals for animals (like humans) or not. It is definitely a good source for plants – and if you sprinkle some in your seed starter mix your plants (depending on the type) may be happy about that (unless your soil is already too alkaline like mine is since I live in New Mexico). But whether humans can absorb the minerals in clay or not...I don't know.

Here's what I can tell you. There was a study that was sponsored by NASA that showed that (at least some) bentonite clay could help support bone density in humans for long term space conditions. That study was what made me initially enthusiastic about bentonite clay for tooth mineralization.

I say there was a study. But I'll be a monkey's uncle if I can find the original paper describing the study. In fact, I can't even find anything at all about the supposed researcher behind the study - Dr. Benjamin Ershoff – other than the numerous mentions in books promoting clay and websites promoting clay. So unfortunately, I cannot verify that any such research actually took place!

Other than that singular supposed study, I can't find any other evidence showing that supplemental bentonite clay is mineralizing for animals. What I have been able to find is that at the very least it does not *de*mineralize with the single exception of iron. Long term supplementation with very large amounts of bentonite clay (5 percent of the diet, which is not something anybody is actually going to do) *may* sometimes reduce iron levels, and increasing iron intake remedies that problem. (Though I suppose if somebody has hereditary hemochromatosis, eating large amounts of bentonite clay *may* be a way to maintain iron levels in range once levels are reduced.)

Although eating clay is often thought of as "far out" when it comes to modern humans, it is mainstream science to study the effects of feeding clay to other animals. The reason is simple: feeding clay to animals has some benefits, including reducing toxic metal burden and detoxifying mycotoxins (toxins from mold, which are found in many foods). (Subramaniam & Kim, 2015)

So the idea of eating clay isn't really all that bizarre and truly does have proven benefits (at least for non-human animals). But all told, I'm no longer convinced that ingesting clay has mineralizing benefits. It *might*. But I just am not convinced.

In case you are interested in ingesting clay, let me add a note. Bentonite clay is primarily made of aluminum silicate. Some people find that scary because aluminum is not something you want to eat a lot of. But it appears that none of the aluminum is absorbed – even with long term feeding. (Elmore, 2003) So that is not a concern.

Finally, bentonite clay is antibacterial and alkaline. When consumed I'm not entirely certain of the implications of that other than the fact that the antibacterial nature can be useful for dysentery. But when used in the mouth, the fact that it is both antibacterial and alkaline means it can reduce tooth decay because it reduces bacteria in the mouth and neutralizes acid that harms teeth.

Ultimately, I am now undecided about the benefits of bentonite clay used internally. I think that for some people it may be beneficial. But I'm not certain enough of the benefits for everybody to recommend it for that purpose.

But it is excellent for rinsing and brushing the teeth in place of harsh, chemical mouthwashes and toothpastes.

In summary, I honestly believe that a few inexpensive supplements can make a big difference. Whereas many people recommend cod liver oil and high-vitamin butter oil that will run you up to $100 per month, I personally find that I get better results from less expensive supplements.

The Thorne D/K liquid can last for many months and works out to just pennies a day. Eating liver and/or supplemental retinyl palmitate is pretty cheap. The gelatin can last for weeks depending on how much you use, and so it is very inexpensive. Likewise with the clay. I purchased a one-pound bag of clay for $16 a year ago, and I am still using it.

Cleaning and Care

I was sick for many years. Very sick. I had chronic Lyme disease, and for several years I could barely even stand up. So I let my tooth cleaning practices go by the wayside. I literally did not brush my teeth for several years.

I tell you this to put things in perspective. I'm not suggesting that it is preferable not to brush your teeth, because I don't feel that way. Now that I can, I do brush my teeth, and I'm glad for it. However, I point this out because many of us have been led to believe that we must brush and floss fanatically or else all our teeth will fall out. The truth seems to be somewhere between these extremes.

As I have already said, I now prefer to brush my teeth rather than not. And, I also enjoy flossing my teeth on occasion. However, I now suspect that brushing and flossing multiple times every day may be detrimental. I think there's a balance to find.

Toothpaste

What I find, and what many other also report, is that brushing and/or rinsing with a "remineralizing" paste is far more effective than using a conventional toothpaste, both in terms of cleaning and improving tooth strength. (I am placing "remineralizing" in quotes because it's not clear whether these pastes actually remineralize directly or not. At least in theory they might since the teeth absorb minerals from saliva.) In fact, many conventional toothpastes include ingredients (such as glycerin) that can interfere with tooth health, so many people find that ditching the conventional toothpastes is a great benefit to their dental health.

Many people have their own preferences for "remineralizing" paste ingredients.

Personally, I like to brush with just water. I find that leaves my teeth feeling clean, fresh, and healthy. On occasion I brush with bentonite clay, which is antibacterial and alkaline – both of which are potentially good for dental health. Also, on rare occasion, I brush with activated charcoal and/or turmeric powder. Beware that both are messy and will stain a toothbrush, porous surfaces, and some dental work (crowns, bridges, possibly some composite fillings?). But on natural teeth both charcoal and turmeric are, somewhat paradoxically, whitening. They are very effective, but I rarely use them because they are so messy.

Other people like to use other ingredients. Some of the most popular ingredients include: baking soda, sea salt, diatomaceous earth, powdered egg shells, coconut oil, and xylitol. Each of these ingredients has potential benefits. Some, such as baking soda and salt, can potentially be irritating to gums over the long run, though plenty of people have been brushing with these ingredients without problems for decades.

Although I personally enjoy brushing with just water or occasionally a small amount of clay, this practice isn't for everybody. Many people are accustomed to using toothpaste, and so they prefer to continue to use something similar. As I have mentioned, conventional toothpastes, even many "natural" toothpastes, include ingredients that may not be good for teeth, including glycerin and things such as sodium lauryl sulfate. These ingredients can prevent teeth from taking in minerals from saliva. So for those who are serious about remineralizing their teeth, it would seem to be best to avoid conventional toothpaste.

You can, of course, make your own "toothpaste" by combining some of the ingredients that I have listed earlier. Many people find that mixing some clay with coconut oil to form a paste is a nice way to do this. And then, because many people enjoy flavored toothpastes, they will add very small amounts of natural 100% pure essential oils (do not use synthetic fragrance oils for this purpose and please beware that essential oils are highly concentrated and not entirely benign) to the toothpaste.

Of course, you may not want to do this yourself. In that case, should you want to get the benefits of a natural toothpaste without having to do it yourself, then you can purchase pre-made products. There are several "remineralizing" toothpaste products on the market. My partner, Sarah, continues to make and sell some of the originals. You can purchase directly from her at:
http://geni.us/rtbshop
Or you can find her products on Etsy
https://www.etsy.com/shop/RowanTreeBotanicals

and Amazon

http://geni.us/rtbamazon

The product containing comfrey root

http://geni.us/comfrey

is intended for short-term use to accelerate tooth healing. For daily, long-term use, consider the remineralizing toothpaste without comfrey root

http://geni.us/toothpaste

Oil Pulling

Oil pulling is another popular technique for mouth care. I have never done this practice daily, though I have experimented with it off and on over the years since I first heard of it back in 2005.

In the previous edition of the book I wrote about my positive experiences with oil pulling. I also was somewhat dismissive of the benefit of using oil specifically versus simply swishing water around in the mouth. But since that time I have done some research into oil pulling, and I can report a bit more on the subject.

It turns out, there are a number of well-designed studies (randomized, double-blind studies) looking at the effects of oil pulling on dental health. One of the clearest benefits is that *regular* oil pulling reduces the count of pathogenic bacteria in the mouth.

Remember that acid-forming bacteria in the mouth are the primary cause of tooth decay. They also form a biofilm called plaque, and that not only contributes to tooth decay (because the plaque is a colony for acid-forming bacteria) – it also can lead to gum disease such as gingivitis.

Therefore, it's not surprising that given its effectiveness in reducing acid-forming bacteria levels in the mouth, oil pulling has positive benefits in terms of reducing and reversing tooth decay as well as gum disease. (Asokan, Emmadi, & Chamundeswari, 2009)

Oil pulling is said to be a traditional Ayurvedic practice going back thousands of years. I can neither confirm nor deny this, though it does seem to be a reasonable claim. It is said that the traditional practice of oil pulling uses sesame seed oil.

I do not believe that it matters what oil one uses, so long as it is a food-safe, non-toxic oil. And it may be that an oil such as coconut oil that has added antibacterial properties may be preferable to sesame oil. The research I've found on the subject has generally used sesame oil, so if you want to replicate the study parameters, use sesame oil. But my partner, Sarah, has found some research showing that coconut oil produced superior results.

In the first edition of this book I suggested that water probably works equally well as oil. But I cannot confirm that is so. All the research uses oil, and I haven't found any research comparing the effects of oil versus water. So again, to replicate the parameters of the research, you'd have to use oil, not water.

The practice is very simple. All you need to do is place a small amount of the oil in your mouth and begin to swish it around. Continue to swish it around for as long as you can stand. Many "experts" suggest that 20 minutes is the ideal. (Now you can understand, perhaps, the inconvenience factor.) Several of the studies I've come across had participants swish the oil for 10 minutes. I don't know if 20 minutes is measurably better than 10 minutes or 5 minutes or 2 minutes since I haven't seen any research comparing the effects of different durations of oil pulling.

As you swish the oil or water in your mouth, you should be sure to swish it between your teeth and around the space between your gums and your lips. The idea is to thoroughly clean your mouth by massaging it with the swishing oil.

Some of the claims for oil pulling are a bit of a stretch, in my opinion. I don't think there is any need to make fantastical claims. It is enough that the practice gives your mouth a thorough cleansing and effectively reduces and reverses tooth decay and gum disease, and if other benefits happen to come along with it, then that is wonderful.

If you feel so inclined, then consider giving oil pulling a try. Many people swear by it. I find it to be quite nice, though I have yet to get in the habit of doing it daily. I find that even once in a while is beneficial. It doesn't necessarily have to be every day. A once a week deep clean is quite lovely. But the research does show that the benefits are cumulative, and the biggest effects show up after 1-2 weeks of daily practice.

You may want to start with plain coconut oil and/or sesame oil. However, my partner, Sarah, also makes an herb-infused coconut oil specifically for oil pulling that you may want to consider. The feedback we receive is very positive. You can learn more about it here: http://geni.us/oilpulling

What Now?

So there you have it - a simple, practical way in which to begin to improve dental health. This information, when put into practice, often helps people to regrow dentin, fill in cavities, improve tooth mineralization, firm up loose teeth, improve receding gums, and more.

Of course, none of this happens magically. You have to actually do it. However, hopefully, I have presented you with a system that is simple to do and easy to maintain. None of this should be particularly restrictive or unpleasant.

So how can you best get started? Well, here's a summary of my recommendations:

First off, understand that your teeth are alive, and as such, so long as the pulp remains intact they can heal when you support them properly (though you are unlikely to be able to regrow lost enamel). The most important thing you can do to support your teeth is to provide your body with enough energy to fuel a healthy metabolism. So if your metabolism is slow, then fuel it with metabolism-boosting food, and lots of it.

Next, without restricting your diet, make sure to add in lots of nutrient-dense foods. Be especially liberal with quality fats such as butter and coconut. Eat lots of quality, mineral-rich food such as dairy, and eat enough quality protein to support growth in your body

Then consider supplementing with fat-soluble vitamins when necessary – vitamins A, K2, and D in particular. I also recommend supplemental gelatin to provide the building blocks for healthy collagen (which makes up to 90 percent of the protein in dentin).

Remember that circulatory health is crucial for dental health. So take care of your cardiovascular system with adequate sleep, sunlight, and movement. In addition, regular consumption of fruits, vegetables, and herbs rich in vitamin C, bioflavonoids, and polyphenols can help to improve circulatory health.

Lastly, ditch harsh toothpastes, and clean your teeth using natural products.

My belief is that all of this is possible to do inexpensively and enjoyably. I sincerely hope that you discover vibrant health, including dental health.

Get Another of My Books for Free

If you've enjoyed this book, there's more where this one came from. And I'd be delighted to give you another one of my books (normally priced at $3.99) for free.

My book *Cleansed* is a reader favorite. Here are some of the things reviewers have to say about it:

> "[G]et the book and enjoy Joey's gift of explaining and educating through the written word"

> "Finally, some sense"

> "This book was worth every minute I spent reading it."

> "I am so thankful to have found and read this book"

Download your free digital copy of *Cleansed* today by visiting http://joeylott.com/cleansed-free-offer

Please Write a Review of This Book

If you liked this book, it would be fabulous if you would write a review of it on site of the retailer from which you got the book

I know, I know. You think it doesn't matter. And it is sort of obnoxious that I ask you to take a minute from your valuable time to do something like write a review of this book.

But actually, reviews are really, really helpful. And that's the reason I ask.

See, the way the retailers work is they help potential readers to discover new books, *but only if those books have* recent *reviews.*

So if you liked this book and would like others to be able to discover it, please do take a moment right now to write a review and post it on the site of the retailer from which you got this book. It really does make a difference.

Thank you.

References

Ashor, A., Lara, J., Mathers, J., & Siervo, M. (2014). Effect of vitamin C on endothelial function in health and disease: a systematic review and meta-analysis of randomised controlled trials. *Atherosclerosis*, 9-20.

Asokan, S., Emmadi, P., & Chamundeswari, R. (2009). Effect of oil pulling on plaque induced gingivitis: a randomized, controlled, triple-blind study. *Indian J Dent Res*, 47-51.

Cass, H. (2013, April 22). *A Practical Guide to Avoiding Drug-Induced Nutrient Depletion*. Retrieved from nutritionreview.org: http://nutritionreview.org/2013/04/practical-guide-avoiding-drug-induced-nutrient-depletion/

Eastoe, J. E. (1955). The amino acid composition of mammalian collagen and gelatin. *Biochem J.*, 589-600.

Elmore, A. (2003). Final report on the safety assessment of aluminum silicate, calcium silicate, magnesium aluminum silicate, magnesium silicate, magnesium trisilicate, sodium magnesium silicate, zirconium silicate, attapulgite, bentonite, Fuller's earth, hectorite, kaolin,. *Int J Toxicol*, 37-102.

Flore, R., Ponziani, F., Di Rienzo, T., Zocco, M., Flex, A., Gerardino, L., . . . Gasbarrini, A. (2013). Something more to say about calcium homeostasis: the role of vitamin K2 in vascular calcification and osteoporosis. *Eur Rev Med Pharmacol Sci*, 2433-2440.

Fox, C., & Eberl, M. (2002). Phytic acid (IP6), novel broad spectrum anti-neoplastic agent: a systematic review. *Complement Ther Med*, 229-234.

Goldberg, M., Kulkarni, A. B., Young, M., & Boskey, A. (2011). Dentin: Structure, Composition and Mineralization. *Front Biosci (Elite Ed)*, 711-735.

Grassi, D., Desideri, G., Giosia, P. D., Feo, M. D., Fellini, E., Cheli, P., . . . Ferri, C. (2013). Tea, flavonoids, and cardiovascular health: endothelial protection. *The American Journal for Clinical Nutrition*, 1660S-1666S.

Holick, M. (2002). Sunlight and vitamin D: both good for cardiovascular health. *J Gen Intern Med*, 733-735.

Iwamoto, M., Yagami, K., Shapiro, I., Leboy, P., Adams, S., & Pacifici, M. (1994). Retinoic acid is a major regulator of chondrocyte maturation and matrix mineralization. *Microsc Res Tech*, 483-491.

Lodish, H., Berk, A., & Zipursky, S. (2000). *Molecular Cell Biology. 4th edition.* New York: W H Freeman.

Lott, J. (2014). *Sleep*. Santa Fe: Archangel Ink.

Lott, J. (2015). *Big Fat Lies*. Santa Fe: Archangel Ink.

Masterjohn, C. (2006, August 2). *Vitamin A On Trial: Does Vitamin A Cause Osteoporosis?* Retrieved from Weston A Price Foundation: http://www.westonaprice.org/health-topics/abcs-of-nutrition/vitamin-a-on-trial-does-vitamin-a-cause-osteoporosis/

Mellanby, M., & Pattison, C. L. (1932). Remarks on THE INFLUENCE OF A CEREAL-FREE DIET RICH IN VITAMIN D AND CALCIUM ON DENTAL CARIES IN CHILDREN. *Br Med J.*, 507–510.

Navneet Singh, c. a., Verma, K. G., Verma, P., Sidhu, G. K., & Sachdeva, S. (2014). A comparative study of fluoride ingestion levels, serum thyroid hormone & TSH level derangements, dental fluorosis status among school children from endemic and non-endemic fluorosis areas. *Springerplus*, 7.

Subramaniam, M. D., & Kim, I. H. (2015). Clays as dietary supplements for swine: A review. *J Anim Sci Biotechnol*, 38.

www.ingramcontent.com/pod-product-compliance
Lightning Source LLC
Chambersburg PA
CBHW060152160125
20473CB00009B/555